W9-BQS-881

Promoting Wellness for Prostate Cancer Patients

MARK A. MOYAD, MD, MPH

CONTENTS

To order Dr. Moyad's, "No B. S. Diet Book" please send your mailing address to
info@annarbormediagroup.com.

All inquiries should be addressed to:
J. W. Edwards, Inc.
2500 S. State Street
Ann Arbor, MI 48104
877-722-2264

Manufactured in the United States of America by Edwards Brothers, Inc.

ISBN-10: 1-930842-04-X
ISBN-13: 978-1-930842-04-5

Third printing, February 2007

WELCOME to a unique educational book for individuals dealing with any aspect of prostate cancer: from prevention to treatment and managing the common (and not so common) side effects of conventional therapy. The goal here is to empower you with lifestyle suggestions and overall information so that you and your doctor or health care professional are better able to communicate and deal with most aspects of this disease.

First and foremost, we thought it would be appropriate to consider potential lifestyle changes that you could use to help prevent heart or cardiovascular disease and potentially improve prostate health. Next, some of the nutritional and dietary supplements that you could take or should avoid are covered. Some attention to bone health is also provided not only because some prostate cancer treatments may cause bone loss, but because the risk of osteoporosis is another concern as individuals get older. In other words, what can you do personally to help combat prostate cancer and possibly improve your general health at the same time? The time seems more than ripe to focus on the forest (general health) over the tree (prostate cancer), because what is the point of treating prostate cancer unless you try to increase your overall chances of living longer and better? There are now more effective treatments available than ever before for all aspects of prostate cancer, and this is the good news that we should never forget. This is also another reason that general health advice should also be a priority—again it is time to focus on the forest over the tree!

The last two chapters of this book contain more prostate-specific information in rapid review. Time seems more precious than ever before; therefore, these chapters are intended to provide a quick "bottom line" review of everything from diagnosis, grading, and staging to treatment, including possible treatment options for treating side effects. These chapters are not intended to replace larger sources of information or other books, but again to improve communication, and to make the most of your visit with your health care professional(s). The last part of this book contains a glossary/dictionary and definitions of some common and not so common words used in prostate cancer.

This book should serve as a general guide to help improve your options and general health, but in the end the decision on what to do or not to do should be between you and your health care professional(s). Thus, this is really a book of suggestions or a map to help guide you in the right direction. It will provide simple tools to use in discussion with your doctor—questions to ask, treatments to consider—to help develop an appropriate strategy to fit your situation. Again, we cannot stress enough that the final decision about what to do or not to do should be between you and your health care professional(s).

Finally, this book is dedicated to you—the individual who is dealing with this disease—and those around you who care for you and support you. You are an inspiration. Your constant requests for more information on this topic helped us to truly recognize the need, and caused us to attempt to satisfy that need in this unique resource. We hope that we have met your expectations.

Mark A. Moyad, MD, MPH
Phil F. Jenkins Director of Complementary & Alternative Medicine
University of Michigan Medical Center
Department of Urology
Ann Arbor, Michigan
Email: moyad@umich.edu

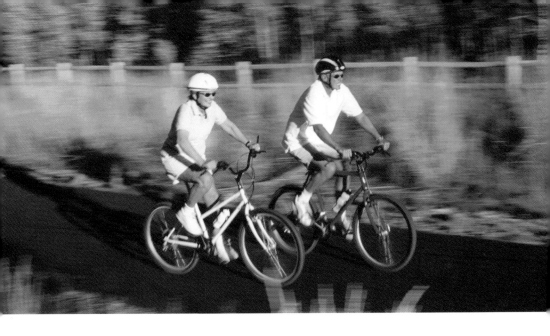

CHAPTER 1: Heart Healthy and Prostate Healthy

Heart disease or actually cardiovascular disease (CVD) is the number one killer of men and women and, in general, what research has shown to be heart healthy has also turned out to be prostate healthy. Since CVD is also the number one cause of death in men diagnosed with prostate cancer, if you become more heart healthy you may get a "2 for 1" effect, so to speak. In other words, now you are doing more to prevent some of the leading causes of early death. Therefore, in this chapter we will look at some ways that you can reduce your risk of developing heart disease and possibly improve prostate health as well.

MONITOR YOUR CHOLESTEROL AND BLOOD PRESSURE

Following a specific prostate healthy diet has never made sense to me because you only have one diet to work with in your daily routine. Since the goal is not just to beat prostate cancer but to live longer and better, the best way to do this is by reducing your chances of dying early from a number of major causes. Therefore, a man should know his cholesterol and blood pressure numbers as well as knowing the results of his latest PSA or prostate exam. One may not be more important than the other. An additional advantage to having your cholesterol measured is that it is a good indicator of how well your lifestyle changes are working. For example, in recent dietary studies of individuals with prostate cancer it should not be surprising that the individuals who followed the healthiest lifestyle programs also had some of the largest reductions in cholesterol.

So, what does a cholesterol test involve? Basically, it measures four things (usually done after fasting for 9 to 12 hours):

Total cholesterol mg/dl	
Less than 200	Desirable
200–239	Borderline high
240 or greater	High

HDL ("good cholesterol") mg/dl	
Less than 40	Low
40–60	Normal
60 or greater	Optimal

LDL ("bad cholesterol") mg/dl	
Less than 100	Optimal
100–129	Near optimal
130–159	Borderline high
160–189	High
190 or greater	Very high

Triglycerides mg/dl	
Less than 150	Normal
150–199	Borderline high
200–499	High
500 or greater	Very high

Other tests such as blood pressure checks or other cardiovascular tests can also be done and should be discussed with your doctor.

Blood Pressure (Systolic/Diastolic)	What does this mean?
Less than 120/80 mm Hg	Normal
120–139/80–89 mm Hg	Pre-hypertensive (moderately high or pre-high blood pressure)
140/90 mm Hg or greater	Hypertensive (high blood pressure)

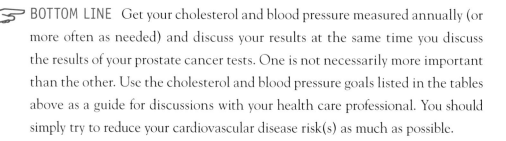 BOTTOM LINE Get your cholesterol and blood pressure measured annually (or more often as needed) and discuss your results at the same time you discuss the results of your prostate cancer tests. One is not necessarily more important than the other. Use the cholesterol and blood pressure goals listed in the tables above as a guide for discussions with your health care professional. You should simply try to reduce your cardiovascular disease risk(s) as much as possible.

MAINTAIN A HEALTHY WEIGHT

Similar to the situation with breast and colon cancer, it seems that maintaining a healthy weight may be one of the most important things individuals can do to not only reduce the risk of cancer, but especially the progression of the disease.

Several of the largest studies ever conducted on this issue have demonstrated that a healthy weight can make a difference after being diagnosed with prostate cancer. Weight is generally measured in a clinical setting by either measuring your body mass index (BMI) or waist-to-hip ratio (WHR).

The BMI chart that follows on page 8 is a quick way to assess your situation, but it does come with one major catch (as does everything in life). An individual who has a lot of muscle mass or begins lifting weights may have a falsely high BMI. This is why the WHR should also be considered. To calculate your WHR, measure your waist at your navel and your hips at the widest point (over buttocks). Divide your waist measurement by your hip measurement. A high number is obviously a concern. The WHR is a good measurement of abdominal or belly size. Discuss these results with your doctor.

Waist to Hip Ratio (WHR)	Health Risk
Less than 0.95	Low risk
0.95-1.0	Moderate risk
Greater than 1.0	High risk

Waist Circumference (WC)
35 to 39 inches = overweight
40 inches or more = obese

 BOTTOM LINE Have your BMI and WHR or just WC measured by your doctor and recorded in your medical chart. The goal is to maintain a normal BMI and WHR or to reduce your weight so that these numbers move more toward a normal range. The chart on page 8 helps you easily find your BMI.

EXERCISE AND MOVE MORE—INCLUDING WEIGHT LIFTING

Does exercise reduce the risk or affects of prostate cancer? Researchers agree that it probably does. We already know that exercise can reduce your risk of numerous cancers and cardiovascular disease, and is one of the best ways to maintain a healthy weight. These facts alone should be enough to motivate you to exercise. An additional benefit is that exercise promotes good mental health as it seems to reduce the risk of depression or recurrence of depression. There are very few things in life that have such a profound impact on both your mental and physical health simultaneously. Wow!

BODY MASS INDEX AND RISKS OF OVERWEIGHT

WEIGHT (lb) →   ← More risk / Less risk

HEIGHT (ft/in)	120	130	140	150	160	170	180	190	200	210	220	230	240	250	260	270	280	290	300	310	320	330
4'5"	30	33	35	38	40	43	45	48	50	53	55	58	60	63	65	68	70	73	75	78	80	83
4'6"	29	31	34	36	39	41	43	46	48	51	53	56	58	60	63	65	68	70	72	75	77	80
4'7"	28	30	33	35	37	40	42	44	47	49	51	54	56	58	61	63	65	68	70	72	75	77
4'8"	27	29	31	34	36	38	40	43	45	47	49	52	54	56	58	61	63	65	67	70	72	74
4'9"	26	28	30	33	35	37	39	41	43	46	48	50	52	54	56	59	61	63	65	67	69	72
4'10"	25	27	29	31	34	36	38	40	42	44	46	48	50	52	54	57	59	61	63	65	67	69
4'11"	24	26	27	30	32	34	36	38	40	43	45	47	49	51	53	55	57	59	61	63	65	67
5'0"	23	25	27	29	31	33	35	37	39	41	43	45	47	49	51	53	55	57	59	61	63	65
5'1"	23	25	27	28	30	32	34	36	38	40	42	44	46	47	49	51	53	55	57	59	61	62
5'2"	22	24	26	27	29	31	33	35	37	38	40	42	44	46	48	50	51	53	55	57	59	60
5'3"	21	23	25	27	28	30	32	34	36	37	39	41	43	44	46	48	50	51	53	55	57	59
5'4"	21	22	24	26	28	29	31	33	34	36	38	40	41	43	45	46	48	50	52	53	55	57
5'5"	20	22	23	25	27	28	30	32	33	35	37	38	40	42	43	45	47	48	50	52	53	55
5'6"	19	21	23	24	26	27	29	31	32	34	36	37	39	40	42	44	45	47	48	50	52	53
5'7"	19	20	22	24	25	27	28	30	31	33	35	36	38	39	41	42	44	46	47	49	50	52
5'8"	18	20	21	23	24	26	27	29	30	32	33	35	36	38	40	41	42	44	46	47	49	50
5'9"	18	19	21	22	24	25	27	28	30	31	33	34	36	37	38	40	41	43	44	46	47	49
5'10"	17	19	20	22	23	24	26	27	29	30	32	33	35	36	37	39	40	42	43	45	46	47
5'11"	17	18	20	21	22	24	25	27	28	29	31	32	34	35	36	38	39	41	42	43	45	46
6'0"	16	18	19	20	22	23	24	26	27	29	30	31	33	34	35	37	38	39	41	42	43	45
6'1"	16	17	18	20	21	22	24	25	26	28	29	30	32	33	34	36	37	38	40	41	42	44
6'2"	15	17	18	19	21	21	23	24	26	27	28	30	31	32	34	35	36	37	39	40	41	42
6'3"	15	16	18	19	20	21	22	24	25	26	27	29	30	31	33	34	35	36	38	39	40	41
6'4"	15	16	17	18	19	21	22	23	24	25	27	28	29	30	32	33	34	36	37	38	39	40
6'5"	14	15	16	18	19	20	21	22	24	25	26	27	28	30	31	32	33	35	36	37	38	39
6'6"	14	15	16	17	18	20	21	22	23	24	25	26	28	29	30	31	32	34	35	36	37	38
6'7"	14	15	16	17	18	19	20	21	23	24	25	26	27	28	29	31	32	33	34	35	36	37
6'8"	13	14	15	16	18	18	19	20	22	23	24	25	26	28	29	30	31	32	33	34	35	36
6'9"	13	14	15	16	17	18	19	20	21	22	23	24	26	27	28	29	30	31	32	33	34	35
6'10"	13	14	15	16	17	18	20	20	21	22	23	24	25	26	27	28	29	30	31	32	34	35

BMI < 25 = Healthy weight
BMI 25–29 = Overweight
BMI ≥ 30 = Obese

$$BMI = \frac{lbs.}{inches^2} \times 704$$

$$= \frac{Kg}{m^2} \quad \left(\frac{\text{weight in kilograms}}{\text{height in meters}} \right)$$

Exercise comes in a variety of forms and you should pick the one that works for you long term. Some people like to walk or walk stairs; others like to swim, row, or use a treadmill or elliptical machine; and others like to garden. Basically, the amount of physical activity you do and the frequency are dependent on your weight. An individual should do enough exercise to help him or her maintain a healthy weight. Some patients have to exercise every day for 30 minutes, while others just exercise 3 or 4 days a week. Obviously, the more active you are the better.

Also, keep in mind that weight lifting is probably as important as aerobic or regular exercise. Weight lifting lowers your risk of osteoporosis, lowers your risk of type II diabetes, helps you to maintain a healthy weight, reduces the risk of heart disease, increases energy levels, and may improve your quality of life.

☞ **BOTTOM LINE** Pick an exercise(s) that you enjoy. The amount of time you exercise should depend on your weight—whatever it takes to maintain a healthy weight is best. Begin to give weight lifting the same importance as aerobic exercise (see chapter 3).

Health Condition	% Reduction with 30 Minutes Exercise/Day
Breast cancer	20–30
Colon cancer	30–50
Depression	25–50
Heart disease	40–50
Osteoporosis	40–50
Premature death	30–50
Stroke	30–50
Type II diabetes	30–40

WORRY MOSTLY ABOUT CALORIES—NOT JUST FAT CONTENT

Just lowering fat intake may not be the answer. Increasing your intake of healthy fats and reducing your intake of unhealthy fats may make more sense. Research in the past has focused on lowering your overall fat intake in order to maintain a healthy prostate. However, recently this has been challenged. Controversy over this issue now exists because it is rather easy today to consume a lot of calories from fat, protein, or sugar. In the past, most calories came from fat, but today portion sizes have changed dramatically so it is easy to get a lot of calories from many sources.

Type of Dietary Fat	Where Is It Commonly Found?	Good or Bad Fat?
Monounsaturated Fat	Cooking oils—canola and olive, Nuts	Good
Polyunsaturated Fat (includes omega-3 fatty acids)	Cooking oils—soy and soybean, and canola, Flaxseed, Fish	Good
Saturated Fat (also known as hydrogenated fat)	Non-lean or high-fat dairy and meats, some fast food	Bad
Trans Fat (also known as partially hydrogenated fat)	Some margarines, fast food, snack foods, deep-fried foods	Bad

The old saying "everything in moderation" really makes sense. Lowering your caloric intake along with regular exercise makes the most sense. There are two types of fat that you should be concerned about—saturated fat, also known as "hydrogenated fat" and trans fat, also known as "partially hydrogenated fat." Both of these types of fat have been linked to heart disease and cancer. Picking up several similar products and choosing the one that is lower in saturated and trans fat is the first step toward healthy eating. For example, when buying margarine, potato chips, or even cookies, try choosing the product that is lowest in saturated and trans fat and also watch that calorie count. Choosing some of the more healthy fats such as monounsaturated and polyunsaturated fats is not only heart healthy, but also seems prostate healthy.

 BOTTOM LINE Calories are the concern and not just fat, protein, or sugar. Consuming smaller portion sizes is the first step toward controlling calories. Good fat and protein sources may also reduce your appetite and increase your HDL. If you are concerned about fat intake, choose items that are low in saturated and trans fat, and increase your intake of monounsaturated and polyunsaturated fat.

NUTRITION LABELS

Do you know how to read a nutrition label? Is the following cholesterol-lowering margarine a healthy product?

Nutrition Facts Serving Size=1 Tbsp.	
Calories 70	Cholest. 0mg
Fat Calories 70	Sodium 110mg
Total Fat 8g	**Total Carb. 0g**
Sat. Fat 1g	Protein 0g
Trans Fat 0g	
Polyunsat. Fat 2g	
Monounsat. Fat 4.5g	

Healthy product—low in calories, high in healthy types of fat (poly- and monounsaturated) and low in the unhealthy types of fat (saturated and trans fat). It is also low in cholesterol, sodium, carbohydrate and protein, which is why it is also low in calories.

How about the following label contents from a popular fast food sandwich?

Nutrition Facts	
Serving Size=1 Sandwich (208g)	
Calories 760	Cholest. 165mg
Fat Calories 430	Sodium 1450mg
Total Fat 48g	Total Carb. 38g
Sat. Fat 20g	Protein Not listed
Trans Fat Not listed	
Polyunsat. Fat Not listed	
Monounsat. Fat Not listed	

Unhealthy product—it is high in calories and high in the unhealthy types of fat (saturated and probably trans fat). It is also high in cholesterol, sodium, carbohydrate and probably protein, which is why it is also high in calories.

BOTTOM LINE Reading nutrition labels or requesting the nutrition information at restaurants is a good way to control calories and decide what is truly healthy and unhealthy for you. Again, talk to your health care professional or a nutritionist for more information on how to read nutrition labels.

INCREASE YOUR INTAKE OF A VARIETY OF FRUITS AND VEGETABLES—NOT JUST TOMATOES

Fruits and vegetables contain many antioxidants and a lot of other so-called anti-heart disease and anti-cancer compounds. In the past, there was a focus on the compound lycopene found in tomatoes for prostate and heart health. However, recent research has focused on a variety of fruits and vegetables and the potential healthful benefits of each. Increasing your intake of a variety of fruits and vegetables will also keep you interested in eating these foods. For example, at our house we like to eat blueberries one day, strawberries on another, broccoli on another, watermelon on another, tomatoes on another, and so on. If we just ate tomatoes every day we would get sick of them in just a few days, and the research does not support this restricted kind of behavior. In fact, watermelon, pink grapefruit, guava, papaya, and other products can contain as much lycopene as a tomato.

Top Sources of Lycopene

-*Tomatoes and tomato products* (ketchup, sauce, soup, powder, paste)

-*Watermelon* (some types actually have more lycopene than tomatoes)

-*Guava*

-*Pink grapefruit*

-*Papaya*

-*Apricots*

BOTTOM LINE Consume a variety of fruits and vegetables daily—not just tomatoes.

CONSUME MORE OMEGA-3 FATTY ACIDS

Omega-3 fatty acids, especially from fish, are not only heart healthy but, you guessed it, they are also prostate healthy. One of the largest medical studies of fish consumption found that eating fish several times a week was associated with a lower risk of advanced or aggressive prostate cancer. Some recent research suggests

Top Sources of Omega-3 Fatty Acids in Fish & Shellfish
(No Fried Fish!!!)

-Mackerel

-Herring

-Salmon

-Cod

-Sardines

-Halibut

-Tuna

-Alaskan king crab

-Anchovies

Top 5 Sources of Soy

-Soybeans

-Tofu or tempeh

-Soy flour

-Soy protein powder

-Miso soup

Top 5 Benefits of Flaxseed Powder over Other Sources of Flaxseed
(oil and pills)

-High in plant estrogens

-High in soluble fiber

-High in omega-3 fatty acids

-Low in calories

-Cheap, cheap, cheap—only costs pennies a day!!!

a lower risk of cancer recurrence after conventional treatment when fish intake was increased.

Eating a variety of fish that is baked or broiled makes sense, but fried fish has not demonstrated the same benefits. Farm-raised and wild fish are both healthy. It seems that as little as 2 servings a week are healthy for you. Tuna fish in a can with water, salmon, cod, and numerous other types of fish are healthy.

There has been a recent concern that some large fish contain high concentrations of mercury, which can be bad for your health. However, this concern is generally for women who are pregnant or trying to get pregnant and young children, and the fish that are of the most concern are king mackerel, shark, swordfish, and tilefish. Otherwise, the positives of eating fish for a healthy heart and prostate far outweigh any negatives for the individuals concerned about getting some mercury. In addition, if you are really concerned about your mercury intake or exposure, you could always ask your doctor about getting a blood test for mercury.

BOTTOM LINE Several servings of fish per week are not just heart healthy, but also prostate healthy. Baked, broiled and even raw fish (sushi) can be healthy, but try to avoid fried fish.

CONSUME MORE PLANT ESTROGEN FROM SOY AND FLAXSEED

The so-called plant estrogens are found in high concentrations in soy and flaxseed products. Both of these products are heart healthy and may reduce your cholesterol. In addition, they are low in saturated and trans fat, high in fiber, and just overall prostate healthy. The Food and Drug Administration (FDA) suggests that 25 grams a day of soy protein from a variety of traditional sources (soybeans, tofu, soy protein powder, and soy milk) may reduce the risk of heart disease along with a reduction in saturated fat intake. Just 1 to 3 tablespoons a day of ground flaxseed is sufficient.

BOTTOM LINE Make soy and flaxseed a part of your regular diet.

LOOK FOR HEART AND PROSTATE HEALTHY COOKING OILS

Cooking oils that are high in monounsaturated fat, high in natural vitamin E, high in omega-3 fatty acids, and lower in saturated and trans fat are not only heart healthy but also seem to be prostate healthy. Oils such as soybean, canola, olive, and safflower are just some of the healthy oils out there. Do not just focus on olive oil because numerous oils are beneficial. However, be careful because 1 tablespoon of any oil contains approximately 120 calories (everything in moderation)!

☞ BOTTOM LINE Utilize a variety of heart-healthy oils in moderation. Read nutritional labels to make sure your oil is high in monounsaturated and polyunsaturated fats and low in saturated fats.

GOING NUTS IS GOOD FOR YOU!

Most nuts are high in vitamins such as vitamin E, high in other antioxidants, low in saturated fat, high in monounsaturated fat, and some even contain omega-3 fatty acids. Also, nuts are a snack that gives you a sense of being full without getting too many calories. It is interesting that nuts such as walnuts, almonds, pistachios, Brazil nuts, and others have been associated with a lower risk of sudden cardiac death and they contain compounds associated with prostate health. For example, Brazil nuts are one of the largest natural sources of selenium, and other nuts are some of the largest natural sources of vitamin E.

☞ BOTTOM LINE Consume a variety of nuts to increase your intake of healthy nutrients and to help control your intake of calories.

CONSUME MORE FIBER—ESPECIALLY SOLUBLE FIBER

Many foods contain a high amount of fiber. Beans, fruits, vegetables, flaxseed, pectin, and oats all contain soluble (viscous) fiber. Also, fiber wafers and powders are a good source of fiber, especially the products that contain a compound called psyllium. These products not only lower cholesterol but they also seem to reduce your risk of a variety of colon problems and may even be prostate healthy. Keep in mind that if you increase your intake of fiber you should also increase your consumption of water, especially when taking a fiber supplement.

☞ BOTTOM LINE Eating 20–30 grams of fiber, especially soluble fiber, a day is a good thing.

Top 5 Reasons to Consume More Nuts

-*High in healthy* (monounsaturated and polyunsaturated) *fats*

-*Low in unhealthy* (saturated) *fats*

-*High in vitamins* (especially natural vitamin E and folic acid)

-*High in minerals* (such as magnesium, potassium, and selenium)

-*High in fiber, protein, and other heart-healthy compounds*

Top 5 Sources of Fiber

-*Beans* (baked, kidney, navy, and lima), *peas or lentils* (legumes)

-*Vegetables* (parsnips, broccoli, brussels sprouts, carrots, and spinach)

-*Fruits* (apple, pear, prunes, raisins, berries, banana, orange, and grapefruit)

-*Breakfast cereals*

-*Nuts, seeds, whole-grain bread and pasta, and brown rice*

MARGARINES AND PRODUCTS WITH PLANT STANOLS/STEROLS MAY BE HELPFUL

There are newer margarines and other products on the market with added compounds called plant stanols or sterols that have been shown to reduce cholesterol and may even be prostate healthy. Talk to your doctor about these government approved margarines to see if you would benefit. They are a little expensive and have to be consumed on a regular basis, but they are healthy. Many of these margarines also contain soybean oil as the active ingredient, so cooking with heart-healthy oils is another option.

☞ BOTTOM LINE Ask your doctor if adding 2 to 3 grams per day of plant stanols/sterols from a couple of tablespoons of such a margarine to your diet makes sense.

WHAT ABOUT DIET PLANS—FADS, MEDITERRANEAN, LOW-FAT, WEIGHT WATCHERS®?

Talk to your doctor or a nutritionist about these diets, but most depend on lowering your intake of calories and exercising more. Regardless, the primary goal is to maintain a healthy weight, cholesterol, and blood pressure and one diet or program does not necessarily work for everyone. Programs like Weight Watchers® are good because they teach you about food, moderation, and portion sizes. An added benefit is that they also involve working with a support group. Low carbohydrate diets may work for some individuals, but long-term they can be difficult to follow. I generally like the Mediterranean diet because it is a moderate and diverse diet with many components. It is flexible, realistic and practical to follow. For example, a typical Mediterranean diet consists of high monounsaturated and low saturated fat intake, moderate alcohol intake, high consumption of bean products and fiber, cereals, fruits and vegetables, and low consumption of meat and meat products, and a moderate intake of milk and dairy products. Basically, this is an "everything in moderation" diet.

Healthy fat and protein sources not only can reduce your appetite, which is a good thing, but may also increase levels of HDL or good cholesterol.

☞ BOTTOM LINE Work with your health professional to find a diet or dietary program that makes sense for you. Keep in mind that if it sounds too good to be true then it probably is. Your health professional should monitor your major numbers including cholesterol, blood pressure, weight loss, and PSA level while you are on a new type of diet just to make sure it is working for you.

ALL OTHER HEART HEALTHY RECOMMENDATIONS MAKE SENSE FOR PROSTATE HEALTH

I could write hundreds of pages on other items that are heart healthy but there are just not enough pages in any book, magazine, or handout to cover all these things in detail. For example, quitting smoking makes sense, not only to reduce your risk of a potentially aggressive cancer, but to increase your chances of living a long life. I am frequently asked if smoking is a clear risk factor for prostate cancer. I generally do not think the association of smoking with prostate cancer even matters because smoking increases your risk of dying early and that should be important enough to make you want to not smoke. Also, smoking has been associated with a lower survival rate in men already diagnosed with many cancers, including prostate cancer. There are so many potential programs and methods to help you quit today that talking with your doctor about these issues makes more sense than ever before.

☞ BOTTOM LINE When in doubt about what to eat or drink or what lifestyle changes to make, just keep in mind that heart healthy equals prostate healthy.

FOCUS ON THE FOREST OVER THE SINGLE TREE

You should also keep in mind one very important thing about lifestyle changes and diet. There is a lot of attention given in the media today about things such as organic versus inorganic fruits and vegetables, artificial sweeteners, caffeine, sugar, chocolate, alcohol, and other changes that may make a difference. However, does reducing or eliminating your intake of these things *really* make a difference? I do not think so. These changes can take the focus off the bigger changes that may truly make a difference. The major changes should really get all the attention, but in reality they sometimes receive little attention. Weight loss, exercise, a moderately healthy diet, reducing blood pressure and cholesterol—these should be receiving the attention. Focusing on your caffeine intake is okay, but only after you take care of the forest before the tree. A checklist of nine moderate lifestyle changes that predicted a 90–95% reduced risk of cardiovascular disease follows on page 16. Can you imagine that! In other words, it is more important to do many things in moderation compared to one or two extremely healthy things.

Yes/No

_____ I don't currently smoke.

_____ I do have "normal cholesterol."

_____ I don't have hypertension.

_____ I don't have diabetes.

_____ I don't have abdominal obesity.

_____ I don't have depression.

_____ I do eat fruits and vegetables.

_____ I don't consume alcohol or drink in moderation.

_____ I do average at least 30 minutes of exercise a day.

Reference: Interheart Study. *Lancet* 364:937-952, 2004.

Please keep in mind that if you have any of the above conditions but they are currently under control (such as depression and diabetes) then you can change your answer to "yes."

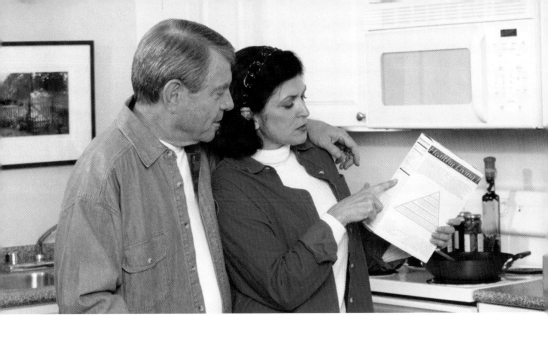

CHAPTER 2: Medications and Nutritional Supplements

Now that you have taken steps to make heart- and prostate-healthy lifestyle changes, you are ready to consider what supplements may be of value to you. We've attempted to provide general information on some of the most common ones considered of use to prostate cancer patients. This information should give you a starting point for discussions with your health care provider on which of the supplements would be good choices for your personal situation. You should always consult with your doctor before starting to take a particular supplement.

When it comes to any dietary supplement I believe less is more and mega-doses are never better. Every individual supplement that I have ever researched comes with serious side effects when taken in mega- or large doses beyond what is truly needed. In fact, many mega-dose supplement studies suggest a worse outcome or prognosis in patients with cancer. In other words, talk to your doctor about whether or not you actually *qualify* for any pill based on your medical history and from the results of your latest medical tests. If you do qualify, talk to your doctor about the precise dose, frequency, and form or brand name of the supplement that was used in the best objective clinical studies that suggested a benefit. This is exactly the same standard doctors use for prescription medications, and dietary supplements should be treated in the same manner.

CHOLESTEROL–, BLOOD PRESSURE–, AND SUGAR–LOWERING MEDICATIONS

The amazing thing about cholesterol-lowering medications is that they not only seem to reduce the risk of cardiovascular disease, but they recently have been associated with better prostate health and may improve your prognosis during and after treatment for prostate cancer. The same findings have been suggested for blood pressure and sugar-reducing (diabetes) medications. This requires further study. If you cannot get your cholesterol, blood pressure, or sugar levels down to normal levels with healthy lifestyle changes, then do not be shy about asking your doctor about some of these medications that may help.

☞ **BOTTOM LINE** Cholesterol-, blood pressure-, and sugar-lowering medications may be prostate healthy. However, even if they are not found to be prostate healthy in the future, they can help to reduce the number one cause of death in men—heart disease.

CHEAP MULTIVITAMINS

In one of the largest and longest studies of cheap multivitamins (Nurses Health Study), women getting a cheap multivitamin over many years with at least 400 mcg of folic acid and 400 IU of vitamin D had a very large reduction in the risk of certain cancers. Recently, a study of men taking a small quantity of a cheap multivitamin also seemed to reduce their risk of dying earlier from all causes. Keep in mind that in most of these studies, individuals were consuming the cheapest multivitamins daily and not expensive ones.

☞ **BOTTOM LINE** A cheap multivitamin that contains selenium, B-vitamins (B_6, B_{12}, and folic acid), and vitamin D seems to be prostate healthy. Check with your doctor on what should be contained in the multivitamin and appropriate amounts for the components.

SELENIUM

In one of the only studies of selenium versus a sugar pill (placebo), selenium supplements (200 mcg/day) were associated with a lower risk of prostate cancer. However, talk to your doctor first about whether or not you should go on an individual selenium supplement. Fish, garlic, Brazil nuts, and numerous other foods contain a lot of selenium. Ideally, a selenium blood test or a toe-nail clippings test (where you actually send toenail clippings to the laboratory—no kidding here) are the best ways to determine whether or not you should go on an individual selenium supplement. The blood test measures selenium intake over the past 2–3 months, and the toe nail clippings test measures your selenium intake over the past 9–12 months (only one of these tests is really needed—talk to your doctor about which one is cheaper and better for you if you are interested in being tested). If the results of your blood or nail clippings selenium test are abnormally low, then one possibility is to first increase consumption of foods that have a lot of selenium. If your selenium levels continue to be low, then the next possibility is to add an individual supplement to your diet. Some multivitamins contain 100 or more micrograms of selenium and this may be enough without having to take an individual supplement.

☞ BOTTOM LINE Increase your consumption of selenium-rich foods. Generally, a cheap multivitamin along with a moderately healthy diet should cover your selenium requirement.

VITAMIN E

Vitamin E supplements, regardless of the dosage, have been very disappointing in terms of their impact on heart disease. In addition, I feel that they have been disappointing so far in terms of reducing the risk or progression of most cancers. In fact, a recent analysis of vitamin E supplement studies suggested that high doses of vitamin E supplements (400 IU/day or more) may actually have no impact on your overall health. Vitamin E supplements can thin your blood too much and they may even reduce the impact of some conventional drugs. However, vitamin E from food may have a positive impact. Vitamin E from food is generally different from the form found in the supplements. In addition, vitamin E in the diet generally comes from a variety of heart-healthy cooking oils, nuts, and seeds.

☞ BOTTOM LINE Ask your doctor if you should take a vitamin E supplement, but keep in mind that most people should not take these individual supplements. There is enough vitamin E in most cheap multivitamins (about 50 IU or 50 mg) to provide what you need. You can also increase your consumption of vitamin E from foods such as heart-healthy oils, nuts, and seeds.

Top 5 Sources of Dietary Selenium

-*Nuts* (especially Brazil nuts)

-*Fish or Shellfish*

-*Poultry or other lean meats*

-*Whole-grain Pasta or Bread*

-*Eggs, garlic, mushrooms, oatmeal, onions and rice*

Top 5 Sources of Dietary Vitamin E

-*Wheat germ oil*

-*Fortified cereals*

-*Heart-healthy cooking oils* (soybean oil, safflower oil, canola oil, olive oil)

-*Nuts* (almonds and others)

-*Seeds* (sunflower seeds and others)

LOW-DOSE ASPIRIN

Low-dose aspirin (81 milligrams) continues to be one of the most promising over-the-counter products (OTCs) to reduce the risk of a variety of conditions. In a very famous recent study low-dose aspirin actually reduced the risk of colon polyps better than regular strength aspirin and caused fewer side effects (internal bleeding and ulcers). In the past few years, low-dose aspirin has been associated with a lower risk of a number of cancers including breast, colon, and prostate cancer, and may even affect the progression of these diseases. In addition, aspirin is heart-healthy because we already know that it can reduce the risk of heart attack. Therefore, if you qualify because of your cardiovascular risk, then you should talk with your doctor about possibly taking a daily low-dose aspirin.

☞ **BOTTOM LINE** Aspirin is not only heart healthy but seems to be very prostate healthy. Please be sure to ask your doctor if you qualify for low-dose aspirin because the side effects of taking aspirin can be very bad. For example, aspirin can increase your risk of an ulcer or a hemorrhagic stroke (internal bleeding).

LYCOPENE SUPPLEMENTS

There have been only a few studies of men taking lycopene supplements for prostate cancer prevention or with conventional treatment and the results thus far are inconclusive and controversial. More studies are desperately needed, but in the meantime if you want to take a low-dose lycopene supplement please talk to your doctor first.

☞ **BOTTOM LINE** We have no idea currently whether or not lycopene supplements reduce the risk or progression of prostate cancer. I am a big supporter of getting more lycopene from food rather than supplements at this time. Regardless, the research is inadequate right now and whether or not you take an individual lycopene supplement at any dosage should be discussed with your doctor.

FISH OIL SUPPLEMENTS

Several studies have suggested that taking fish oil pills containing the two primary fish oils, EPA and DHA, (500 mg–1 gram per day) may reduce the risk of sudden cardiac death and may reduce the risk of other cardiovascular events. In addition, fish oil may reduce triglycerides, which may be increased in men on some treatments for prostate cancer, and may have anti-arthritic and anti-cancer properties as well as other important benefits. Fish oil pills also tend to be low in mercury. However, keep in mind that even fish oils come with a catch. They may thin your blood too much and increase your risk of internal bleeding. Please discuss with your doctor whether or not you qualify for a fish oil supplement. Obviously, individuals already on another blood thinning medication have to be careful when combining it with fish oil pills.

☞ BOTTOM LINE Fish oil pills are heart healthy for some individuals and may also be prostate healthy. However, first talk to your doctor about whether or not you qualify for this supplement because in some individuals these pills may thin your blood too much.

FIBER SUPPLEMENT

This was discussed earlier, but potentially taking a daily fiber supplement can improve your cholesterol numbers and may reduce the risk of gastrointestinal problems. First, talk to your doctor to see if you qualify for a daily fiber supplement such as psyllium or modified citrus pectin, or another fiber pill, powder, or wafer.

☞ BOTTOM LINE A daily inexpensive fiber supplement may not only improve your cholesterol numbers, but also may impact PSA and reduce your risk of gastrointestinal problems. You should always drink a glass or two of water with every fiber supplement.

CALCIUM AND VITAMIN D (ALSO SEE SECTION ON OSTEOPOROSIS)

Calcium and vitamin D supplements are not only heart healthy, but also seem to be colon healthy, bone healthy, and may even be prostate healthy. Talk to your doctor about whether or not you need to take these supplements. Calcium carbonate (antacid supplements) has been well studied, but other calcium supplements such as calcium citrate and calcium phosphate may work as well. Vitamin D from supplements may also be an additional option but, in reality, the vitamin D blood test is a very accurate way to determine whether or not you need a supplement.

☞ BOTTOM LINE Talk to your doctor about whether or not you qualify for calcium and vitamin D supplements. Also, the vitamin D blood test is a great test to determine how much vitamin D you need. This test ideally should be done in the fall or winter when vitamin D levels in the body are the lowest.

OTHER SUPPLEMENTS

Please keep in mind that most other dietary supplements are not needed at this time. If you are interested in a unique dietary supplement, you should discuss it with your health care provider.

IMPORTANT NOTE:

Please keep in mind that I generally advise that 2–3 weeks before any surgical or radiation procedure patients should discontinue the use of almost all dietary supplements. Preliminary evidence has demonstrated that some supplements may thin your blood during surgery, may interact with the anesthetic used in surgery, or may reduce the impact of radiation or other conventional treatments. Therefore, in order to be safe rather than sorry, it is best to focus on healthy lifestyle and dietary changes during this time. When you have recovered from surgery or have completed radiation or other conventional treatments, then you and your doctor should discuss when it is okay to restart the use of certain dietary supplements. This general rule should also apply to chemotherapy or other treatments. Always have a discussion with your doctor before conventional prostate cancer treatment begins about which supplements are and are not appropriate during this time. However, again less is more when it comes to dietary supplements during conventional prostate cancer treatment. There will always be exceptions to this general rule. For example, some doctors advise vitamin D supplementation with some chemotherapy drugs and others do not. Again, as always, the ultimate decision about which dietary supplements to discontinue or maintain during conventional prostate cancer treatment should be between you and your doctor. Regardless, it is always beneficial to focus on healthy lifestyle changes during the time of conventional treatment (see Chapter 1).

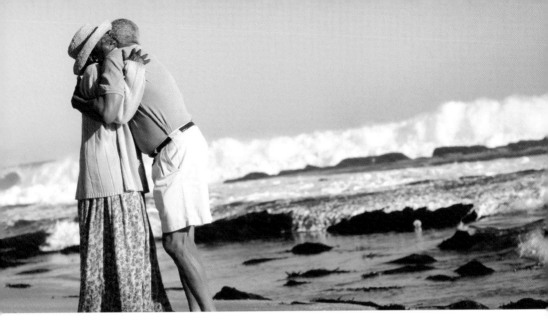

CHAPTER 3: Bone Health

Bone health is not only an issue with some testosterone reducing treatments for prostate cancer, but it is fast becoming a serious concern for men in general as they get older. In fact, although bone health and bone fractures are much more common in women than men, it is now an accepted medical fact that men have a greater chance of dying from a bone fracture compared to women. Therefore, bone health has also become a major men's health issue similar to the concern we expressed earlier over cardiovascular disease risk. There are no symptoms until a bone fracture occurs so we need to consider how to prevent this from happening in the first place. We will discuss some of the common risk factors of bone loss or osteoporosis (including testosterone reduction). Then, we will discuss how it is diagnosed. Finally, we will discuss how to prevent bone loss through lifestyle changes and possibly medications for some individuals.

STEP 1. CONSIDER THE POTENTIAL RISK FACTORS FOR OSTEOPOROSIS OR BONE LOSS

Read the list below and discuss those factors that are relevant to you with your doctor.

• Advanced Age—Aging is one of the biggest risk factors. As we get older, the bones can become weaker due to a number of factors, including lower testosterone levels.

- Alcohol intake (excessive)—Alcohol in excess can cause bone-building cells in the body to become less effective. In moderation, alcohol may lower the risk of bone loss due to its estrogenic effects. If you drink alcohol, please always drink in moderation, 1 to 2 servings of alcohol per day. (Note: A serving of alcohol is twelve ounces of beer, 4–6 ounces of wine, or 1.5 ounces of liquor.)
- Caucasian or Asian race—African Americans in general have a lower risk of osteoporosis, but other men tend to have a higher risk.
- Drugs—Anticonvulsants, LHRH agonists and antagonists, glucocorticoids (also known as "steroid" drugs), certain blood thinners (long-term use), NSAIDs, long-term use of some pain medications, and certain thyroid medications.
- Endocrine disorders
- Family history/genetics—Risk increases with the number of family members affected by osteoporosis and certain genetic mutations.
- Gastrointestinal diseases
- Genetic and metabolic diseases
- History of a previous fracture—Increases risk for another fracture
- Low sunlight exposure—Getting little or no sunlight can reduce the body's level of vitamin D, and vitamin D is needed to protect your bones. Only 10 to 15 minutes of sunlight (ultraviolet B waves) exposure two times a week without sunscreen activates the production of vitamin D by the body.
- Neoplastic conditions or other cancers
- Neurologic diseases
- Propensity for falls or risk factors that increase your risk of falling and suffering from a fracture—Postural instability or a lack of proper posture that can increase the risk of falling, neuromuscular impairment, poor vision, lower limb weakness, drugs that affect blood pressure, lack of precautions in household and other surroundings, etc.
- Pulmonary diseases
- Renal diseases
- Sedentary lifestyle, immobilization, or lack of weight-bearing exercise—Lack of exercise, especially a lack of resistance and impact exercises (weight lifting) can increase risk.
- Small body frame or low weight—Obesity may actually reduce the risk of osteoporosis and fracture due to increased conversion of testosterone to estrogen in adipose (fat) tissue. Estrogen can also protect your bones.

- Smoking—Tobacco smoke may alter hormone levels and suppress bone-building factors.
- Surgery to remove the testicles (orchiectomy).
- Transplantation bone disease
- Vitamin and mineral deficiency—Low intakes of elemental calcium and vitamin D, deficient diet or lack of supplementation, and possibly low intake of boron, vitamin K, and other vitamins and minerals in the diet.
- Vitamin and mineral excess—(excessive intakes of vitamin A and D) can actually inhibit the cells in the body needed to make more bone—so again, everything in moderation.

STEP 2. UNDERSTAND HOW CLINICIANS DIAGNOSE OSTEOPOROSIS.

An imaging (picture) test is used to help determine the status of your bone health. There are numerous imaging tests that a doctor may use and these are discussed in Step 3. An imaging test usually takes a picture of one or several sites of the body and it compares your picture or bones to that of a 25- to 30-year-old male, the benchmark age range where individuals have the optimal bone health. If your bone or bones are similar to the benchmark then this is considered normal. If your bones are a little less dense or a little weaker than the benchmark, this is called osteopenia. Osteoporosis is when your bones are much weaker than the benchmark. Finally, if you have already had a fracture and your bones are much weaker than a young person's, then this is called severe osteoporosis. The weaker your bones are compared to a young person's, and the more bone loss you have experienced, the more likely that you will experience a fracture in the future unless intervention occurs that reduces your risk of continued bone loss.

STEP 3. LEARN ABOUT THE DIFFERENT SCREENING, DETECTION, OR IMAGING MACHINES

There are numerous devices available today to help a doctor determine whether your bones are normal, osteopenic, or osteoporotic. The section that follows will give you basic information on the commonly used imaging tests. You should discuss them with your physician to determine which would be most appropriate for your situation.

I would make several general recommendations for your consideration before and after having a bone density screening.

Recommendation #1: If possible, always have your imaging tests done at the same location, with the same machine, and same health-care professional to reduce error.

Recommendation #2: Always ask the health care professional at the test site if the device is comparing your bones to those of a man or a woman. Ideally you want them compared to those of a man.

Recommendation #3: Always ask for a copy of your results from the imaging tests and for a copy of the recommendations as a result of your test. Keep in mind that some individuals may get a test result that says that they have bones that are normal, osteopenic, and osteoporotic all at the same time because the multiple bones tested (hip, spine, and wrist) may be in differing conditions.

Recommendation #4: Make sure you understand the out-of-pocket and insurance-covered costs of the tests.

Now it is time to review all the different imaging tests that are used to evaluate bone health. Please review the information below with your doctor before deciding which test is right for you.

SCREENING TESTS FOR OSTEOPOROSIS

Dual-Energy X-ray Absorptiometry (DEXA) (Recommended for most men)
• Fairly inexpensive; low-radiation exposure; rapid and easy to perform. Is the accepted "gold standard" for detecting/diagnosing osteoporosis. It also is the most multiple site specific test (spine, hip, wrist). Newer software also allows for an accurate determination of body fat.
• Osteoarthritis of the lumbar spine and/or aortic calcifications falsely elevate this measurement in older patients. Ask your doctor if you have any of the conditions that could increase your chances of a false finding.

Heel Ultrasound (HUS) (Not recommended for most men)
• Cheap, rapid, easy to perform in an office setting; low risk to the patient. May assess the initial risk for fracture.
• Lacks overall sensitivity (up to 10% false-negative rate). Whether or not this indirect anatomical site provides direct evidence is controversial. Additionally, little information is known about the accuracy of having several measurements over time. Should only be used initially to decide if a patient is at risk for a fracture. Any follow-up imaging tests should be performed with another device (DEXA or QCT).

Quantitative Computerized Tomography (QCT) (Recommended for some men when a DEXA is not adequate)

- Most sensitive method available to detect osteoporosis of the spine.
- Expensive; high-dose radiation exposure for the patient

X-ray (plain radiograph) (Not recommended to determine bone health in men with prostate cancer)

- Routine use in a variety of fields of medicine may help to indirectly determine whether or not there is a great deal of bone loss at some body sites.
- Not generally utilized because bone losses of 40–50% are required to detect an abnormality.

Other Newly Developed Imaging Tests—peripheral DEXA (p-DEXA), peripheral QCT (p-QCT), radiogammetry (Not recommended for most men)

- Rapid, inexpensive, and safe. May assess the initial risk for fracture.
- Similar to HUS, these devices measure an indirect site (finger, heel) to decide what may be occurring at a more direct site. They should only be used to access initial risk. Any follow-up or treated patient should be tested with a more conventional device (DEXA or QCT). Also, minimal research has been completed with these devices compared to conventional scanners.

STEP 4. UNDERSTAND THAT THE PROPER EVALUATION OF BONE HEALTH MAY INVOLVE MULTIPLE TESTS.

Imaging tests are the best single way to evaluate bone health. There are additional or ancillary tests that help to provide the most complete and accurate evaluation. Your doctor will consider your history, perform a physical exam, and possibly recommend other laboratory tests (blood and urine).

STEP 5. UNDERSTAND THE IMPORTANCE OF THE VITAMIN D BLOOD TEST.

It is important to talk about one blood test specifically that is fairly inexpensive and may tell you and your doctor about your risk of a future fracture. This is the vitamin D blood test. Normal blood levels of vitamin D are needed to maintain proper bone health. There are two vitamin D blood tests, but the first test, 25-hydroxy-vitamin D, is the more adequate test for most patients. However, the second test may also be used in patients with abnormal kidney function. Either way, this test helps clinicians determine whether or not you have

The best way to determine your vitamin D requirement is to simply get a vitamin D blood test.

an adequate amount of vitamin D in your body, and whether or not you need to get more vitamin D from a variety of sources. Ask your doctor about getting this test and keep in mind that the test is most accurate when it is done in the late fall or winter time because this is when vitamin D levels tend to be the lowest (due to less ultraviolet B light exposure from the sun). However, the test can be done any time of the year.

Many individuals need to increase their intake of vitamin D because it increases the absorption of calcium and so helps to improve bone health. In general, doctors recommend that you get between 400 and 800 IU of vitamin D daily from a variety of sources. However, some doctors may want you to get even more than 800 IU of vitamin D if the results of your tests suggest that you need more.

SOURCES OF VITAMIN D

• Fortified beverages and foods—Milk, soy, protein bars, cereal, and a variety of other beverages and foods are fortified with vitamin D. Check the label on the product to determine the amount.

The only foods that naturally* contain vitamin D are:

-*Eggs* (small source=25 I.U. in one egg)

-*Mushrooms* (small source=50 I.U. per serving)

-*Seafood* (the largest natural source=100 to 500 I.U. per serving in most healthy fish/shellfish)

*(otherwise foods and beverages need to be fortified with this vitamin)

• Fish and fish oils—Fish and some fish oil supplements contain a high level of vitamin D. Be careful with some supplements because they may also contain very high levels of vitamin A, which can be bone unhealthy.

• Multivitamin (cheap) or an individual vitamin D supplement—Most contain at least 400 IU of vitamin D.

• Prescription drugs—Calcitriol and other vitamin D sources can be prescribed and taken orally or given as an injection if the doctor thinks you need to get vitamin D from these sources.

• Sun (ultraviolet B light) 10–15 minutes of sunlight several times per week especially during the spring and summer allows the human body to make vitamin D. Sunscreen users, African Americans, overweight, and older individuals have a more difficult time making this vitamin.

STEP 6. UNDERSTAND THE IMPORTANCE OF GETTING CALCIUM FROM A VARIETY OF HEALTHY SOURCES.

Men generally need to have a total daily intake of 1000 to 1500 milligrams of elemental calcium from food and beverages and/or supplements. The specific amount of calcium intake needs to come from your doctor. Some men need more calcium and others need less depending on the results of their tests. Ideally, keeping a weekly food and beverage intake diary can help you and your doctor determine how much calcium you are getting from your diet.

Now, the bad news—much of the calcium that you get from food or beverages is not completely absorbed by the body. When determining the amount of calcium intake needed with your doctor, keep in mind that only about 33–50% of the total calcium from food and beverage sources is actually absorbed. This will help you do the proper math when adding up your total calcium intake. This may sound a little frustrating, but you can easily reach your calcium goal by also getting some additional calcium from a supplement (see step 7).

Calcium Rich Foods

-*Collard greens*
-*Orange juice* (fortified)
-*Sardines*
-*Oatmeal* (instant)
-*Yogurt*
-*Milk*
-*Figs* (dried)
-*Cheese*
-*Nuts*

STEP 7. UNDERSTAND THE SIMILARITIES AND DIFFERENCES BETWEEN CALCIUM SUPPLEMENTS

There are a variety of different calcium supplements available on the market today. The good news is that, regardless of the cost, they are all quite effective, and they all can make it much easier to reach your total daily calcium intake goal. The bad news is that depending on which calcium supplement that you and your doctor choose, there are different requirements when taking them. The table that follows will give you some considerations to discuss with your doctor in determining which calcium supplement might be the best choice for you.

Calcium supplements should be taken in divided doses because the human body generally absorbs approximately 500 mg of elemental calcium at a time. Check for the amount of "elemental calcium" in each tablet because this is the form of calcium that is absorbed and actually counted for the required daily calcium intake for women and men. Some of the above supplements may also contain vitamin D, increasing the tablet size. If tablet size is a concern, get your vitamin D from a separate source. In addition to improving bone health, calcium and vitamin D may have a very positive affect on a number of other health concerns as well as improving dental health. It just makes good sense to get an adequate supply of calcium and vitamin D in your diet or from supplements.

Similarities and Differences between Some Over-the-Counter Calcium Supplements	
Supplement	Brand name
Calcium carbonate (contains 40% elemental calcium) These supplements are usually inexpensive. Should be taken with food because you need some stomach acid to absorb them. Older individuals and those on proton pump inhibitor (PPIs) drugs and on chronic antacid drugs will have a more difficult time absorbing calcium from these supplements.	Caltrate OsCal Rolaids TUMS Viactiv Oyster shell calcium Coral calcium Generic brands
Calcium citrate or calcium citrate malate (contains 21% elemental calcium) Can be taken with or without food. Probably the preferred form for those with a history or risk of oxalate kidney stones, but if you are worried about a kidney stone, you should take this supplement with meals.	Citracal Generic brands
Calcium phosphate (contains 39% elemental calcium) Can be taken with or without food	Posture-D Generic brands

STEP 8. WEIGHT-BEARING OR RESISTANCE EXERCISES TO IMPROVE BONE HEALTH

No individual should begin a weight-lifting program without the approval of a doctor and the help of a professional trainer. Some men with very weak bones and those men who have cancer in their bones or other serious conditions may not be good candidates for weight-lifting exercises. Again, check with your doctor to see if you can start a weight-lifting program.

The benefits of lifting weights are very remarkable. Recent research in men has demonstrated that lifting weights just 2 to 3 times per week can:

Improve bone health and reduce osteoporosis risk.

Reduce your risk of falls and injury.

Reduce fatigue and increase energy levels.

Improve overall quality of life.

Improve cardiovascular health.

Improve insulin sensitivity and reduce diabetes risk.

Reduce body fat and discourage excess weight gain.

Improve your mood.

Wow! Weight training can really do a lot for any man. Talk to your doctor about the possibility of starting a weight lifting program. Some of the suggested weight-training exercises that were used in a large study of men (Segal, R. J. et al, *J Clin Oncol*, 2003) are listed below in the table and can be used as a discussion topic for you, your doctor, and a professional trainer in order to get started. You may choose to do these exact exercises, or your doctor and trainer may suggest modifying these a bit. Men in the weight-lifting study did these nine exercises three times a week. It only takes about 30 to 40 minutes to accomplish all nine of these exercises.

Weight lifting exercises were shown in a recent study to improve the lives of men with prostate cancer in just 12 weeks.*

Exercise	Initial reps	Additional reps (plus 5 lbs of weight)
Leg extension	12	8
Calf raises	12	8
Leg curl	12	8
Chest press	12	8
Latissimus pull-down	12	8
Overhead press	12	8
Triceps extension	12	8
Biceps curls	12	8
Modified curl-ups	12	8

*Note: Some doctors or trainers also like to include a back lift in order to strengthen the spine. A small or low weight that is shaped like a small sac or cushion or bag (just a few pounds) is placed on the upper back and lying on your stomach you do 8 to 12 push ups. This places resistance on the spine and may improve bone mineral density in this area.

STEP 9. UNDERSTAND THE VARIETY OF DRUG TREATMENTS FOR BONE HEALTH AND THEIR ADVANTAGES AND DISADVANTAGES.

Only your doctor can decide whether or not you need to be on a drug for bone health. Keep in mind that with any drug treatment, the recommended intakes of daily vitamin D and calcium and other lifestyle changes still usually apply because these increase the effectiveness of the drug therapies. Also keep in mind that drugs called "bisphosphonates" are still the gold standard or preferred treatment for bone loss. Bisphosphonate drugs come in a pill and injection form. Also, keep in mind that most of the drug treatments for bone health do not impact or reduce hot flashes (with estrogen being the one exception). You should discuss all of the drug options available to improve bone health with your doctor to decide if you need medication and which drug would most improve your situation.

Any man, and not just those on testosterone lowering treatment, should discuss bone health and maintaining bone health with their doctor. Getting older is simply one of the biggest risk factors for bone loss.

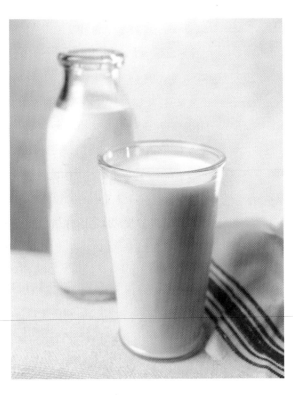

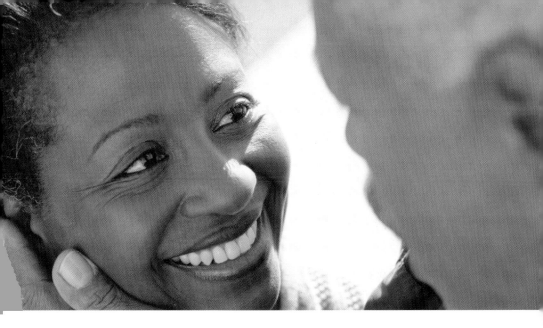

Chapter 4: From Diagnosis to Grading (aggressiveness of your cancer) to Staging (location of your cancer)

This chapter is simply a quick guide to be used with your doctor in terms of discussing anything from the anatomy of the prostate gland to biopsy to grading and staging. It is a summary to help you better understand your prostate cancer and how it is acting and where it may be located. *Please use this material with your physician.*

THE ANATOMY OR LOCATION OF THE PROSTATE GLAND

Notice that the prostate sits deep in the pelvic area of the body (Figure A, page 34). It consists of 3 zones: the peripheral zone or PZ (65–70% of the total area of the prostate), the central zone or CZ (20–25% of the total area of the prostate), and the transition zone or TZ (5–10% of the total area of the prostate). Most prostate cancers begin growing in the PZ, and this is the area or zone that can be felt by the doctor during the digital rectal exam (DRE). The DRE only takes seconds. Prostate cancer less frequently grows in the CZ and TZ, but the TZ surrounds the urethra or part of the body that carries urine from the bladder to the penis. The TZ is where Benign Prostatic Hyperplasia (BPH or non-cancerous enlargement of the prostate) occurs, which is also common and can cause urinary problems. *Please discuss with your health care professional the specifics of prostate anatomy.*

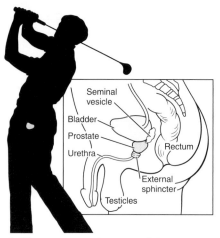

Figure A. The anatomy or location of the prostate gland.

THE PROSTATE BIOPSY

Keep in mind that for most individuals it is impossible to diagnose prostate cancer unless you have a prostate biopsy (Figure B). The doctor will take numerous samples (also called "cores") from a variety of the different areas of the prostate. These samples are sent to a pathologist who will read them and decide whether each and every sample taken has normal cells, cancer cells, or something that is not cancer but is also not quite normal in appearance. For example, High-Grade Prostatic Intraepithelial Neoplasia (HGPIN) may increase the risk of you having cancer in a future biopsy. HGPIN is not cancer, but it is not normal either. Also, if you have been diagnosed with cancer the pathologist that looks at your slides will attempt to determine how aggressive your cancer is (also called "grading") and also try to determine if your cancer is contained within the prostate or has spread beyond the prostate (also called "staging"). *Talk to your doctor about the results or possible results of your biopsy. We recommend that, as with most other medical information, you especially request a copy of the results of your biopsy for your own records.*

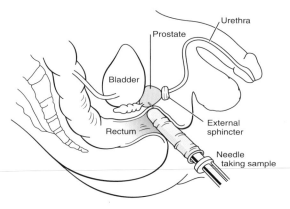

Figure B. The prostate biopsy.

Here is a summary of the potential Gleason scores that could appear on your
pathology report (Table 1). Keep in mind that every single prostate biopsy sample
with cancer will be assigned its own Gleason score, but overall please discuss
what your overall Gleason score means with your doctor. In general, the lower
your Gleason score the less aggressive the cancer, and the higher the Gleason
score the more aggressive the cancer. However, a lot of information from your
pathology report is used to determine the overall aggressiveness of your cancer.
For example, an individual with a low Gleason score, but with a lot of cancer in
most of the samples may need to also be treated aggressively just because there is
so much cancer in the prostate.

Table 1 - Possible Gleason Scores	
Gleason Scores	**What Does that Tell Us?**
1+1, 2+1, 1+2, 1+3 2+1, 2+2 3+1	2–4 = Well differentiated cancer or not aggressive
1+4, 1+5 2+3, 2+4 3+2, 3+3 4+1, 4+2 5+1	5–6 = Moderately differentiated cancer or moderately aggressive
2+5 3+4 4+3 5+2	7 = Moderately poorly-differentiated or aggressive
3+5 4+4, 4+5 5+3, 5+4, 5+5	8–10 = Poorly differentiated cancer or very aggressive

Please discuss with your doctor where your cancer has spread based on this system (Tables 2, 3, and Figure C on pages 36–38). This is a difficult system to have any book explain and it is really best to have your doctor show you where on this system your cancer is, and what this means to you. Keep in mind that numerous tests and not just the pathology report can be used to determine the specific location of your cancer.

		TABLE 2 — The ABCD and New TNM Clinical Staging Systems for Localized Prostate Cancer
ABCD	**TNM**	**What Do the Results Mean?**
—	TX	The cancer cannot be staged at this time.
—	TO	There is no evidence of a cancer.
A	T1	A cancer that cannot be felt with a DRE or picked up by an imaging machine (X-ray, CT scan, MRI, etc.) or is found by PSA or another procedure, such as a TURP for BPH. This is "localized or confined prostate cancer."
A1	T1a	A cancer that is found during a procedure such as a TURP (not found by a biopsy). The cancer takes up less than 5% of prostate tissue removed in the procedure.
A2	T1b	A cancer that is found during a procedure such as a TURP. The cancer takes up more than 5% of the prostate tissue removed in the procedure.
B0	T1c	A cancer that cannot be felt with a DRE but it is detected by a biopsy in one or both sides of the prostate, because of an initial high PSA level.
B1 or B2	T2	The cancer is only confined or within the prostate, and/or it has invaded the apex of the prostate (where the urethra leaves the prostate), or it has gone into but not beyond the prostate capsule. This is still called a "localized or confined prostate cancer."
B1	T2a	A cancer that occupies only one side (lobe) of the prostate.
B2	T2b	A cancer that occupies both sides (lobes) of the prostate.

TABLE 3 — The ABCD and New TNM Clinical Staging Systems for Advanced Prostate Cancer

ABCD	TNM	What Do the Results Mean?
C1–C2	T3	The cancer goes through the prostate capsule. This is also called "locally advanced prostate disease."
C1	T3a	A cancer on one or both sides of the prostate that is now growing on the outside and going beyond the prostate. This is also called "unilateral (one side) or bilateral (both sides) extracapsular extension."
C2	T3b	A cancer that has invaded one or both seminal vesicles.
C2	T4	A cancer that has spread to or invaded other nearby structures other than the seminal vesicle(s) such as the: bladder neck, external sphincter, rectum, nearby muscles (also called "levator muscles") and/or the pelvic wall. This is also called a "locally or regionally advanced prostate cancer."
—	NX	The lymph nodes cannot be staged at this time.
—	NO	No lymph nodes near the prostate have cancer (or metastasis). These are also called "regional lymph nodes."
D1	N1	Cancer in a regional node or nodes near the prostate. This is also called a "regionally advanced prostate cancer."

Note: The regional lymph nodes are in the pelvic area and there are 5 sets of them called: Pelvic, Hypogastric, Obturator, Iliac, and Sacral.

ABCD	TNM	What Do the Results Mean?
—	MX	Metastasis or cancer spread far beyond the prostate (also called "distant metastasis") cannot be staged at this time.
—	MO	There is no metastasis or cancer spread far beyond the prostate (also called "no distant metastasis").
D2	M1	Cancer has metastasized or spread far beyond the prostate (also called "distant metastasis"). This is also called "Advanced Prostate Cancer."
D2	M1a	Cancer has metastasized or spread to a node or nodes far beyond the prostate (also called "nonregional lymph node or nodes").
D2	M1b	Cancer has metastasized or spread to the bone or bones.
D2	M1c	Cancer has metastasized or spread to another site or sites in the body far beyond the prostate (such as the liver, lungs, and bones). This is the most advanced category or stage of prostate cancer.

Note: The nonregional lymph nodes are far from the prostate and there are 8 sets of them called: Aortic (also called "para-aortic lumbar"); Common iliac; Inguinal; Superficial inguinal (also called "femoral"); Supraclavicular; Cervical; Scalene; and Retroperitoneal.

Note: M or Metastasis, or cancer spread far beyond the prostate commonly goes to a bone or bones. In addition, during metastasis, the cancer can commonly go to nonregional or distant lymph nodes. Prostate cancer to the lung is uncommon with metastasis but when it occurs it usually is because it has gone along the distant lymph nodes to eventually reach the lung. Liver metastasis or cancer that has spread to the liver is very uncommon and it usually occurs late in the course of this disease.

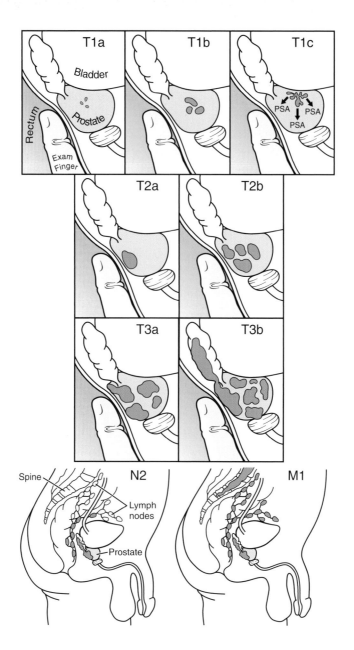

Figure C. The progression of prostate cancer, from the earliest stages to the most advanced, along with the corresponding TNM and ABCD stages.

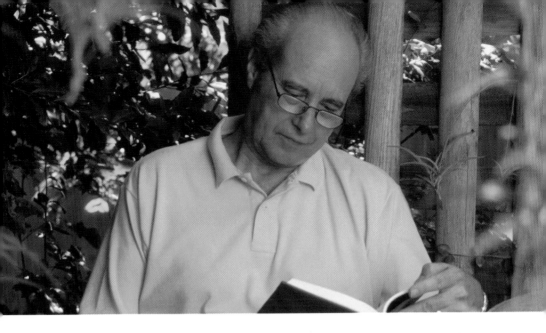

Chapter 5: Treatment Options and Treating Side Effects

Please use this chapter in a similar way that you used chapter 4. It is simply a quick review of the various treatment options for prostate cancer. There are a whole range of treatment options available today from simple active surveillance (watchful waiting) to localized treatments to hormone treatments to chemotherapy to clinical trials. This chapter is included to help you and your doctor understand some of the more popular treatment options and how to reduce some of the side effects. Also, please discuss with your doctor a list of the potential advantages and disadvantages of each treatment. The goal here is not to advise you on the best treatment, but to enhance the communication with your doctor when deciding which treatment is best for you. Some patients may have more than one of these treatments. For example, some men get radiation and/or hormone therapy if the PSA rises after surgery.

SURGERY

The incisions (Figure A) and step-by-step order in which the surgeon carries out the radical prostatectomy procedure (Figure B), and the final reconstruction involved in the surgery (Figure C) are shown in the illustrations that follow. The average total time for a radical prostatectomy is 2–3 hours. Keep in mind that some doctors also offer a laparoscopic surgery or robotic surgery and this should also be reviewed with the doctor.

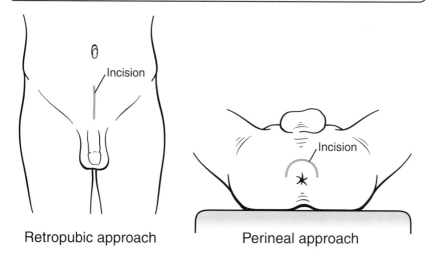

Incision types

Incision

Retropubic approach

Incision

Perineal approach

Figure A. The incisions used in the two types of radical prostatectomy.

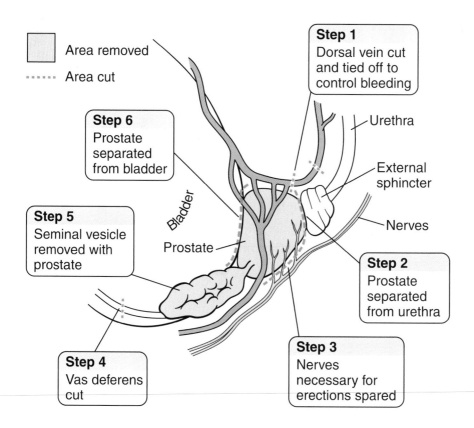

Area removed

Area cut

Step 1
Dorsal vein cut
and tied off to
control bleeding

Urethra

Step 6
Prostate
separated
from bladder

Step 5
Seminal vesicle
removed with
prostate

Bladder

Prostate

External
sphincter

Nerves

Step 2
Prostate
separated
from urethra

Step 4
Vas deferens
cut

Step 3
Nerves
necessary for
erections spared

Figure B. The prostatectomy procedure.

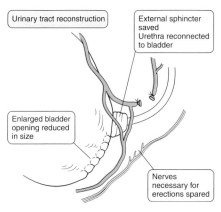

Figure C. The reconstruction.

RADIATION THERAPY

There are a number of radiation therapies, most commonly including external-beam radiation treatment (EBRT), brachytherapy, and temporary radioactive-seed implantation. External-beam radiation therapy is delivered from an external source outside the body to the prostate to kill the cancer and stop it from growing (Figure F, page 42). This treatment requires coming to the hospital five days a week for four to six weeks, with each treatment session lasting about 15–30 minutes.

Brachytherapy is another type of radiation delivered from inside the body, in which radioactive seeds or pellets that emit radiation are implanted in order to kill the surrounding tissue including the cancer (Figure D). Before the seeds are implanted in the prostate, a great deal of time is spent understanding exactly where the cancer is and the precise location of the prostate. There are different

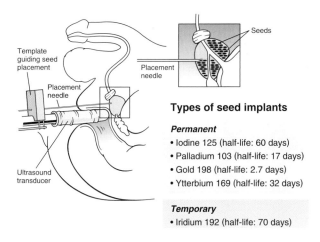

Figure D. A side view of permanent radioactive-seed implantation performed under the guidance of transrectal ultrasound, or TRUS.

types of radioactive seeds that may be used, with Palladium-103 and Iodine-125 being the most common. The procedure takes one to several hours.

Temporary radioactive-seed implantation involves placing an intense radiation source directly in or around the cancer for a short period of time. Done under ultrasound guidance, 12–20 small, flexible plastic needles are inserted through the perineum and into the prostate (Figure E). This procedure requires a short stay in the hospital.

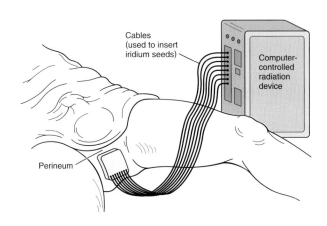

Figure E. Temporary radioactive-seed implantation: Iridium seeds (also called "bars") are inserted and timed using a computer-controlled radiation device.

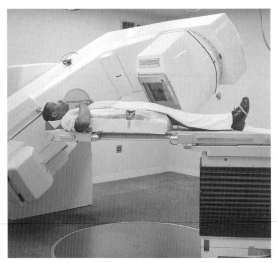
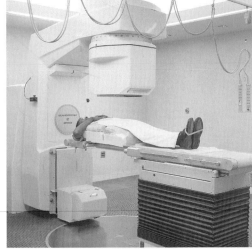

Figure F. External-beam radation therapy.

CRYOSURGERY

During cryosurgery (Figure G), several supercooled probes are inserted through the perineum (the area between the anus and scrotum) into different areas of the prostate. A warmer may also be used to reduce side effects. A transrectal ultrasound probe (covered with a condom) is inserted into the rectum to help guide the procedure. When the probes are removed, each of the punctures requires only a single suture, or stitch, to close. Keep in mind that some doctors are also using cryosurgery today for men with a prostate that have a rising PSA after radiation treatment.

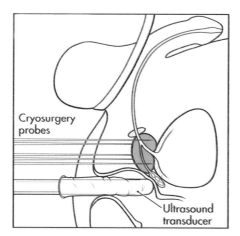

Figure G.
Side view of the cryosurgery procedure.

RECURRENCE

Below is a sample of some of the issues involved in predicting disease recurrence. Keep in mind that many nomograms, or risk charts, exist today for predicting the actual risk of your cancer returning after localized treatment. Pleases discuss any nomograms or prediction tables with your doctor. Issues include:

Preoperative PSA	Surgical Margins
Gleason Sum	Seminal Vesicle Invasion
Prostatic Capsule Invasion	Lymph Nodes

SIDE EFFECTS

Treating the various side effects of localized prostate cancer treatment should be discussed with your doctor. For example, a discussion of incontinence treatment is beyond the scope of this book because there are so many options. However, we have included a summary of potential treatments for erectile dysfuncion, as well as a broad discussion of treatments for hot flashes, and these are listed below.

A partial summary of treatments for erectile dysfunction (E.D.) (Table 4). Keep in mind that in some men more than one treatment can be used.

Table 4 - Treatment For Erectile Dysfunction (E.D.)		
Type of Therapy	Advantages	Disadvantages
Oral medication phosphodiesterase inhibitors (also known as "PDE-S inhibitors")	• Pills taken by mouth • Effective for most men	• Not effective in patients who have had prostatectomy, unless some nerve-sparing approach was used • Side effects include headache, blurry vision, joint or back pain • Should not be used in some patients • 30–60 minutes wait for response • Cannot be taken with some medications
Intra-urethral suppository	• Small pellet placed in the urethra without needles • Few systemic side effects • Effective in some men	• Can cause penile pain • Requires training • Refrigeration required • May require tension ring placed at base of penis for best effects • Side effects include (rarely) painful and prolonged erection of more than six hours, fainting, dizziness
Penile injection	• Highly effective • Few systemic side effects • Works in three to five minutes	• Some medications require refrigeration • Requires injection • Requires office training • Can cause penile pain • Can cause prolonged erection and penile scars or fibrosis
Vacuum device	• Least expensive • No systemic side effects • Effective in most patients	• Can cause numbness or bruising • Less "natural" erection • Trapped ejaculate • May be awkward to use
Penile prosthesis	• Highly effective • For men who have failed or are not satisfied with medical treatment of impotence	• Small risk of infection • Requires anesthesia and surgery • May require replacement after many years of use

Reference: University of California San Francisco Medical Center, *Managing Impotence—A Patient Guide*, N. Rahman, S. Rosenfeld, T. Lue, and P. Carroll, 2005.

Testosterone reducing treatment is used in a variety of situations and should be discussed with your doctor. Table 5 lists the common and not so common side effects of hormone reducing or manipulation treatment. Please discuss how to prevent or reduce any of these side effects with your doctor.

Table 5 - Side Effects of Lower Testosterone	
Side Effect	**What This Actually Means**
Anemia	Blood less able to carry oxygen to supply energy to body cells
Cholesterol changes	May increase cholesterol levels especially due to weight gain
Cognitive impairment	Unable to remember things; a feeling of mental fogginess
Depression, mood changes	Feeling sad or listless, uninterested in life
Edema	Swelling due to water gain, especially in legs
Fatigue	A feeling of being tired all the time
Genital atrophy	Shrinking of penis and scrotum
Gynecomastia	Growth or enlargement of breasts; pain or tenderness in breasts
Hair changes	Loss of body hair, increased scalp hair
Erectile dysfunction/loss of libido	Inability to get or maintain an erection/feeling uninterested in sex
Hot flashes	Sudden feeling of heat; may last seconds or minutes at a time
Muscle atrophy	Loss of muscle and strength
Musculoskeletal pain	Pain in muscle and joints
Osteoporosis or osteopenia (bone loss)	Weak bones; increase in risk for fractures
Thyroid problems	Changes in level of thyroid hormone (usually reduced)
Weight gain	Gain of non-muscle weight, especially in the belly or waist area

HOT FLASHES: WHAT WORKS AND WHAT IS WORTHLESS?

When your level of testosterone is reduced, one of the most common side effects is hot flashes or hot flushes, and they can be mild, moderate, or even severe. It is difficult if not impossible to predict who will experience hot flashes, how often, and how severely. Thus, we decided to include information on defining and treating hot flashes. If you follow the steps in this section, you will become more familiar with how serious your hot flashes are and whether or not they should be treated by conventional or alternative treatment, or if they should just be left alone. Let's get started.

UNDERSTAND THAT HOT FLASHES MAY OR MAY NOT REQUIRE TREATMENT

In hot flash clinical trials, most patients responded to some type of minimal intervention, but some patients can experience hot flashes that do not respond to simple lifestyle changes. For most mild to moderate hot flashes a prescription drug is not needed, but for moderate to severe hot flashes a prescription drug is usually needed. Keep in mind that many of the hot flash remedies do not address the potential bone loss that may occur with androgen deprivation treatment (see chapter 3 on bone health).

Before deciding with your doctor about the proper treatment for your hot flashes, you need to determine the frequency and severity of the hot flashes.

DEFINE THE FREQUENCY AND SEVERITY OF YOUR HOT FLASHES

Keep in mind that the duration is not necessarily as important as your discomfort level. For example, some severe hot flashes may last less than a minute but cause a disruption of work or sleep. Conversely, some hot flashes will last for several minutes but will not cause you to sweat or change your behavior. These should still be considered a mild hot flash. The table on the following page will help you with your evaluation.

Severity of hot flash	Score	Duration	Discomfort
Mild	1 Point	Less than 1 minute	Warm & slightly uncomfortable, no perspiration
Moderate	2 Points	Less than 5 minutes	Warmth involving more of the body, perspiration, removing layers of clothing
Severe	3 Points	Greater than 5 minutes	Burning warmth, disruption of normal life activities such as sleep or work, excessive perspiration, thermostat changes

Reference: Moyad, M. A. "Moyad Hot Flash Scale." *Urol. Oncol.*, 2005.

TRACK YOUR HOT FLASHES

Be sure to photocopy the following hot flash diary several times to enable tracking for multiple weeks.

PERSONAL HOT FLASH DIARY

Name _____

Week Starting _____

	Hot flashes per day			Points			Total number of flashes	Total points	Activities increasing or decreasing hot flashes
	Mild	Moderate	Severe	Mild (1 pt each)	Moderate (2 pts each)	Severe (3 pts each)			
Mon									
Tue									
Wed									
Thu									
Fri									
Sat									
Sun									
Summary for the Week									

Weekly Average Hot Flash Intensity Score: _____

(Divide weekly points by total number of hot flashes)

Other Observations: _____

_____

_____

DISCUSS POSSIBLE TREATMENT OPTIONS WITH YOUR DOCTOR

Using your Hot Flash Diary pages as a discussion tool, your doctor can help you develop appropriate treatment options. By determining the average severity of the problem and by quantifying the disruption to your daily activity, your health care professional can work with you on a suitable plan to help alleviate the hot flashes. You may also begin to notice certain activities or food and beverages that affect the number and severity of the hot flashes, either positively or negatively, and begin to adapt your habits to improve the situation.

TREATMENT OPTIONS FOR HOT FLASHES

There are a variety of treatments for hot flashes. Please review them with your doctor.

Alternative remedies and lifestyle changes

Examples include acupuncture, flaxseed, soy, paced respiration, wearing loose clothing, ice cubes (see "More Information" for more details). These may help with mild to moderate hot flashes, however, more testing is needed. Some may not be helpful or may be harmful, so talk to your doctor about the latest research. The impact on bone mineral density is not known and probably minimal.

Medications

Your doctor may suggest different types of prescription medications for your hot flashes.

Other new potential agents

Check with your doctor for the latest information on new therapies.

MORE INFORMATION ON ALTERNATIVE REMEDIES AND LIFESTYLE CHANGES FOR HOT FLASHES

Let's take a look at some of the potential alternative remedies and lifestyle changes that may help relieve mild to moderate hot flashes. Keep in mind that many of these have not been well studied and should not be used without consulting your physician.

Acupuncture (via electrostimulation)

Maybe. Potentially effective, but has not been tested against placebo. A few studies suggest that 1 to 2 acupuncture treatments a week may reduce hot flashes.

American or Asian Ginseng (Panax quinquefolius or Panax ginseng)

No. Has not worked and may significantly lower blood sugar levels.

Beta-sitosterol (phytosterol)

No. Not adequately tested yet, but it is a component in some approved cholesterol-lowering margarines.

Bioflavonoids (fruit juices and skins)

No. Not tested yet.

Black cohosh (Cimicifuga racemosa)

Maybe. May reduce sweating symptoms, but awaiting more trial results. Also, may abnormally increase liver enzymes.

Blue cohosh (Caulophyllum thalictroides)

No. Not adequately tested yet.

Chinese Herbal Combinations

No. Not tested yet or has not worked.

Chasteberry (Vitex agnus castus)

Maybe. Has been beneficial for PMS symptoms for women so may help some men.

Dong quai (Angelica sinensis)

No. Has not worked in clinical studies.

Evening Primrose Oil (Oenothera biennis)

No. Has not worked in clinical studies.

Flaxseed (Linum usitatissimum)

Maybe. Has worked in some studies, and may lower cholesterol levels. Flaxseed powder is the most researched form. (See chapter 1 for heart-healthy information on flaxseed.)

Hops (Humulus lupulus)

No. Not adequately tested yet.

Licorice root (Glycyrrhiza glabra)

No. Some effectiveness possible, but may increase blood pressure in some men.

Oregano (Origanum vulgare)

No. Not adequately tested yet.

PC-CALM, PC-SURE, and other PC- products (mixture of herbs, some are estrogenic)

No. Not adequately tested yet and may contain enough estrogenic material to cause a blood clot.

Red Clover (Trifolium pratense)

Maybe. Caution needed as some products may contain coumarins that could cause abnormal blood thinning.

Resveratrol (3,4',5-trihydroxystilbene from grapes and wine)

No. Not adequately tested yet.

Saint John's wort, SAM-e

Maybe. Be careful because they may reduce the effectiveness of some prescription drugs.

Soy (Glycine max)

Maybe. Minimal impact with supplements, but possible impact with traditional dietary sources such as soybeans and soy protein powder. May lower cholesterol.

Thyme (Thymus species)

No. Not adequately tested yet.

Turmeric (Curcuma longa)

No. Curcumin may have anti-cancer affects and may lower cholesterol, but additional testing is needed.

Verbena (Verbena species)

No. Not adequately tested yet.

Vitamin E (tocopherols and tocotrienols)

No. Alpha-tocopherol has not worked better than placebo and may be harmful in dosages of 400 IU or more. Other natural sources of dietary vitamin E (gamma-tocopherol) have not been tested.

Wild Yam (Dioscorea villosa)

No. Topical supplements have minimal benefit in initial studies.

OTHER PRACTICAL OPTIONS

A number of lifestyle changes including low-impact exercise; stress reduction; paced respiration; avoiding hot beverages; using ice cubes, cool beverages, and fans; wearing loose clothing; and reducing room temperature may provide symptomatic relief. Talk to your doctor and continue to keep a hot flash diary to see which changes may provide most relief to you.

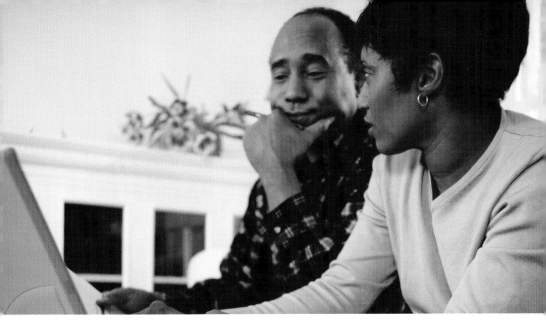

Glossary

Abdominal-Pelvic CT (computed tomography) Scan

An abdominal-pelvic CT (computed tomography) scan is an X-ray scan that images the various organs in the abdomen and pelvis. It is used to determine whether the pelvic lymph nodes have been affected with prostate cancer.

Adjuvant Therapy

Adjuvant therapy is an additional treatment used to increase the effectiveness of the primary therapy.

Adrenal Androgens

The adrenal glands, which sit on top of the kidneys, produce small amounts of male hormones (androgens), including testosterone. While about 95% of testosterone is produced by the testicles, about 5% to 10% comes from the adrenal glands. The effect of adrenal hormones on prostate cancer is unknown. Some physicians think they can contribute to the spread of prostate cancer while others think that the quantity is not large enough to be of concern. (On the other hand, there is no question that testosterone from the testicles can increase the growth rate of prostate cancer.)

Alkaline Phosphatase

Alkaline phosphatase is an enzyme in blood, bone, kidney, spleen and lungs. An alkaline phosphatase test is used to detect bone or liver metastasis.

Alpha-Blockers

Alpha-blockers are drugs that act on the prostate by relaxing certain types of muscle tissue. These drugs are often used in the treatment of BPH, but not in the treatment of cancer.

Androstenedione

(also known as "Andro") This is a dietary supplement as well as a compound that is made naturally by the human body. Most men on androgen suppression should not take the supplement because it can be converted to testosterone and also can reduce your levels of HDL (good cholesterol).

Antiandrogen

An antiandrogen is a compound (usually a synthetic pharmaceutical) that blocks or otherwise interferes with the normal action of androgens at cellular receptor sites. It is often used with an LHRH agonist.

Antiandrogen Withdrawal Response (AAWR)

Antiandrogen withdrawal response (AAWR) is a decrease in PSA caused by the withdrawal of an antiandrogen after combined hormonal therapy (CHT) begins to fail. It occurs when there are PCa cells that have mutated to feed on the antiandrogen rather than on testosterone (T) or dihydrotestosterone (DHT).

Anticholinergic Drugs

Anticholinergic drugs are medications that can be used to treat urinary incontinence.

Artificial Sphincter

An artificial sphincter is an implantable device used to treat urinary incontinence (loss of urinary control) that has persisted for a long time.

AST (SGOT)/ALT (SGPT)

A blood test that helps to determine whether or not your liver is functioning properly. Some doctors like to use this test routinely to determine if a drug (such as a cholesterol-lowering drug) or supplement is impacting your liver function.

Benign

Benign is relatively harmless; not cancerous; not malignant.

Benign Prostate Hyperplasia (BPH)

Benign prostate hyperplasia (BPH) is a noncancerous condition of the prostate that results in the growth of tissue, enlarging the prostate and obstructing urination.

Bone Scan

A bone scan is a technique more sensitive than conventional X-rays that uses a radio-labeled agent to identify abnormal or cancerous growths within or attached to bone. In the case of prostate cancer, a bone scan is used to identify bony metastases that are definitive for cancer that has escaped from the prostate. Metastases appear as "hot spots" on the film. However, the absence of hot spots does not prove the absence of tiny metastases. Bone scans can also be positive because of old injuries or arthritis.

Bowel Preparation

Bowel preparation is the cleaning of the bowels or intestines, which is normal prior to abdominal surgery such as radical prostatectomy.

Color-Flow Doppler Ultrasound (CDUS)

Color-flow Doppler ultrasound (CDUS) is an ultrasound method that may image tumors more clearly by observing the Doppler shift in sound waves caused by the rapid flow of blood through tiny blood vessels that are characteristic of tumors.

Combination Hormone Blockade (CHB)

Combination hormone blockade (CHB) is the same as combined hormonal therapy (CHT) or androgen deprivation therapy (ADT) or maximal androgen blockade (MAB). It usually involve an LHRH agonist and an antiandrogen.

Combined Hormonal Therapy (CHT)

Combined hormonal therapy (CHT) is the use of more than one kind of hormonal therapy.

Computed Tomography Scan

Computed tomography scan is also called a CT, or CAT, scan. This involves a large number of X-rays which, when stacked together, provide a three-dimensional, cross-sectional view of certain structures in the body. It helps some doctors with prostate-cancer staging. It also can assist in more accurate delivery of external-beam radiation by determining the exact position of the prostate.

Computerized Axial Tomography

Computerized axial tomography (also known as CT scan and CAT scan) is a method of combining images from multiple X-rays under the control of a computer to produce cross-sectional or three-dimensional pictures of the internal organs, which can be used to identify abnormalities. It can identify prostate enlargement, but is not always effective for assessing the stage of prostate cancer. However, for evaluating metastases of the lymph nodes or more distant soft tissue sites, the CAT scan is significantly more accurate.

Conformational Therapy

Conformational therapy is the use of careful planning and delivery techniques designed to focus radiation on the areas of the prostate and surrounding tissue that need treatment and to protect areas that do not need treatment. Three-dimensional conformational therapy is a more sophisticated form of this method.

CPK (Creatine phosphokinase)

(or CK Creatine kinase) A blood test used to measure muscle function. High scores on the test could indicate muscle problems. It is standard to monitor the results of this test for many individuals on a variety of drug treatments, especially cholesterol-lowering medications.

Creatinine
A blood test used by some doctors to measure kidney function. This is a standard blood test for individuals on most drug therapies and one monitored in those being treated with a drug for bone health.

DHEA & DHEAS
A supplement as well as a compound made in the human body that can be converted into testosterone. Most men on androgen suppression should not take this supplement because it can increase testosterone levels.

DVT
(Deep Venous Thrombosis) A DVT is a blood clot that usually occurs in the veins of the legs. It can detach and go to the lungs. Some medical conditions and treatments for cancer, such as estrogen treatment or estrogen-like drugs, and some supplements can cause this dangerous condition.

Fat
(or body fat) Can be concentrated in the body in two forms—subcutaneous fat that accumulates under the skin and visceral fat that occurs deeper in the body around the organs. Visceral fat is the bigger concern of the two because it can cause numerous health problems. Reducing testosterone can increase your levels of fat in the body, especially subcutaneous fat. To reduce the risk of accumulating excess body fat, every man on testosterone reduction treatment should also be on an exercise program and some should include weight lifting.

Fatigue
The general feeling of being tired or having a lack of energy despite an adequate diet and sleep pattern. This can be caused by a number of drug treatments. There are simple treatments for fatigue such as exercise and weight lifting and drug treatments for more serious forms of fatigue.

Five-alpha-Reductase Inhibitors
Five-alpha reductase (5-alpha-reductase) inhibitors are a type of drug that prevents the conversion of testosterone to dihydro-testosterone (DHT). These drugs are used to help treat BPH.

Homocysteine
A blood test used by some doctors in addition to a basic cholesterol test. This test may give added information to help establish your risk of cardiovascular disease. High levels of this blood marker may be associated with a higher risk.

Also, high levels may be associated with a greater risk of other conditions such as neurological disease and bone loss. Higher intake of some B-vitamins (B_6, B_{12}, and folic acid) may reduce abnormally high levels of homocysteine. However, keep in mind that this is still a controversial test.

Hormone-Dependent vs. Hormone-Independent Prostate Cancer

Hormone-dependent cancer needs hormones from the body to grow and live. If someone has prostate cancer it is better to have the hormone-dependent variety, because today's treatments can shut off the hormone production that fuels cancer growth. Hormone-independent cells, on the other hand, can thrive without the presence of hormones—they will continue to grow regardless of whether the hormone supply is cut off. Therefore, some other type of treatment other than hormonal therapy (chemotherapy) is needed to try to stop these cells from growing.

Hot Spots

Hot spots are images on a bone scan that indicate where prostate cancer has spread to the bones.

hs-CRP

(High-sensitivity C-Reactive Protein) Another blood test used by some doctors in addition to a basic cholesterol test. This test may give some added information to help establish your risk of cardiovascular disease and possibly other conditions. Many of the lifestyle changes and drug therapies that reduce cholesterol or improve cardiovascular health can reduce abnormally high levels of hs-CRP. This is an inexpensive test, but is still a somewhat controversial test.

Insulin

(or Insulin Resistance) Insulin is a compound released by the body in response to increases in blood sugar levels. Insulin helps with the uptake or absorption of sugar into the body. High levels of insulin are associated with a number of unhealthy conditions. Some men may experience an increase in insulin due to an increase in body fat and reduction in muscle tissue. Generally, a man should have his insulin levels checked periodically and should eat a healthy diet, exercise, and potentially lift weights to reduce abnormal levels of blood insulin.

Intermittent Androgen Blockade (IAB)

A type of hormonal therapy in which hormone therapy is cycled on and off over a period of months to try and decrease the side-effects of hormonal therapy.

Kegel Exercises

Kegel exercises are exercises designed to improve the strength of the muscles used in urinating.

Libido

(also known as sexual desire or sexual drive) This is a condition that should be discussed with your doctor. You and your doctor should decide how much your libido is impacted by certain treatments and what to do if it occurs. Most men with a reduced libido can still have an erection and orgasm.

Magnetic Resonance Imaging (MRI)

Magnetic resonance imaging (MRI) is the use of magnetic resonance with atoms in body tissues to produce distinct cross-sectional, and even three-dimensional images of internal organs. MRI is primarily of use in staging biopsy-proven prostate cancer.

Metabolic Syndrome

A condition or a series of abnormal numbers that have been associated with a greater risk of some health conditions. Some men should discuss ways to reduce this problem with their doctor. An individual with at least three of these five conditions is at risk for metabolic syndrome.

- Abdominal obesity: waist circumference greater than 40 inches (102 cm)
- Triglycerides greater than or equal to 150 mg/dL
- HDL less than or equal to 40mg/dL
- Blood pressure greater than or equal to 130/85 mmHg
- Fasting glucose greater than or equal to 110 mg/dL

Musculoskeletal Pain or Discomfort

A general feeling of pain or tenderness in a certain group of muscles or throughout the body. It has been reported in a small number of patients on a variety of drug therapies for prostate cancer. Some doctors simply follow this condition because it can improve with time. Some doctors treat it with vitamin D because it can indicate a deficiency. Still other doctors may do additional testing and other treatments for this problem if it comes from a more serious condition such as cancer or tumor growth in the bones.

Prostatectomy

Nerve-sparing radical prostatectomy is an operation to remove the prostate that allows at least one of the two nerve bundles near the gland to be saved. Sparing these nerves greatly increases a man's chance of retaining normal sexual function.

Palliative Treatment

Palliative treatment is designed to relieve a particular problem without necessarily solving it. For example, palliative therapy is given in order to relieve symptoms but does not provide a cure.

Positron Emission Tomography (PET)

Positron emission tomography (PET) uses a radioactive isotope that is taken up by tumor tissue to show that the tumor is functional. Current studies do not indicate a high utility of PET scanning in prostate cancer that is newly diagnosed, perhaps related to the usual slow doubling times.

PSA (free)

A free PSA assay, reports the percentage of free-PSA to total-PSA (total PSA = free PSA + bound PSA). It is helpful for screening purposes when PSA values are above the normal threshold for an age group (greater than 4), but less than 10. One study showed that men with PSA ratio >25% had no PCa; those with <10% were likely to have PCa.

PSA Density

PSA density is a formula used to determine a man's chances of having prostate cancer and thus the need for a biopsy. It involves dividing the PSA value (in ng/ml) by the volume, or size, of the prostate (based on transrectal ultrasound).

PSA Velocity

PSA velocity is the change in PSA level over time. The currently accepted normal annual PSA increase is 0.75 ng/ml. PSA velocity is particularly useful in monitoring two types of men: those whose PSA level is increasing rapidly but is still within the normal range, and those with a suspiciously high PSA level who have normal biopsy results.

Saw Palmetto

A popular alternative medicine used to provide some relief for the symptoms of benign prostate enlargement.

Spot Radiation

Spot radiation is external-beam radiation treatment for bone pain that is associated with advanced prostate cancer. Radiation targeted to painful areas of bone does not stop the cancer from growing, but it can help ease some of the pain.

Three-Dimensional Treatment Planning and Conformal Therapy

Three-dimensional treatment planning and conformal therapy is a type of external-beam radiation therapy that uses computerized images from a CT scan to help precisely conform the radiation beam to the shape of the tumor. This allows the delivery of the most powerful dose of radiation to the prostate while minimizing the risk of damage to surrounding structures.

Transrectal Ultrasound (TRUS)

Transrectal ultrasound (TRUS) is a diagnostic procedure that uses echoes of ultrasound waves (far beyond the hearing range) to image the prostate by inserting an ultrasound probe into the rectum; commonly used to visualize prostate biopsy procedures.

Transrectal Ultrasound (TRUS)-Guided Biopsy of the Prostate

Transrectal ultrasound (TRUS)-guided biopsy of the prostate is a prostate biopsy that is performed under the guidance of transrectal ultrasound, in which sound waves from a rectal ultrasound probe act as a navigator to let the doctor accurately locate the prostate for tissue sampling. A tiny needle is then inserted alongside the probe to remove a small sample of prostate tissue.

Watchful Waiting

Watchful waiting is when a man diagnosed with prostate cancer decides to carefully monitor the progress of his cancer rather than opting for immediate treatment. This is an active process that involves the man and his doctor.

Zinc

A mineral that has been promoted as a prostate-healthy supplement. High levels of zinc intake from supplements (for example 100 or more milligrams per day) can be associated with abnormal immune changes, a reduction in the effect of bone-building drugs, abnormal changes in the cholesterol blood tests, and may even be prostate unhealthy. Most men on androgen suppression do not need to get more than 20 milligrams of zinc per day from supplements (ideally as part of a cheap multivitamin) unless instructed otherwise by your doctor.

Resources for Patients and Caregivers

ADVOCACY AND SUPPORT ORGANIZATIONS

American Cancer Society
www.cancer.org
(800) ACS-2345

American Society of Clinical Oncology
www.asco.org

American Urological Association
www.auanet.org

CancerCare
www.cancercare.org
(800) 813-HOPE

Foundation for Cancer Research
and Education (FCRE)
www.cancer-foundation.org
(434) 974-1303

MaleCare
www.malecare.com
(212) 673-4920

Man to Man, local groups of the
American Cancer Society
www.cancer.org
(800) ACS-2345

National Comprehensive Cancer
Network
www.nccn.org

National Prostate Cancer Coalition
www.pcacoalition.org
(888) 245-9455

Patient Advocates for Advanced
Cancer Treatments
www.paactusa.org
(616) 453-1477

Prostate Cancer Education Council
www.pcaw.com
(866) 477-6788

Prostate Cancer Foundation
www.prostatecancerfoundation.org
(800) 757-CURE

Prostate Cancer Research and
Education Foundation
www.pcref.org
(619) 461-8181

Prostate Cancer Research Institute
www.prostate-cancer.org
Helpline: (800) 641-PCRI

Prostate Forum
www.prostateforum.com

The Prostate Net
www.prostate-online.org
(888) 477-6763

Us TOO International Prostate Cancer
Education and Support Network
www.ustoo.org
Support hotline: (800) 808-7866
(800) 80-Us-TOO

GOVERNMENT AGENCIES

The Centers for Disease Control (CDC)
www.cdc.gov/cancer/prostate

National Cancer Institute (NCI),
a division of the National Institutes
of Health (NIH)
www.cancer.gov
www.nci.nih.gov/cancertopics/types/
prostate
(800) 4-CANCER

National Center for Complementary and
Alternative Medicine (NCCAM), a division of the National Institutes of Health
(NIH)
www.nccam.nih.gov
(888) 644-6226

National Library of Medicine, a division of
the National Institutes of Health (NIH)
www.nlm.nih.gov

OTHER RESOURCES

American Institute for Cancer Research
www.aicr.org

American Pain Foundation
www.painfoundation.org

Association of Cancer Online Resources
www.acor.org

Consumerlab.com, LLC. A quality control
site offering the best quality health and
nutrition products through independent
testing
www.consumerlabs.com

Erectile Dysfunction Information Center
www.cure-ed.com

HRPCa.org. Developed by and for patients
with hormone-refractory prostate cancer;
frank, well-researched, patient-centered
information
www.hrpca.org

National Family Caregivers Association
www.nfcacares.org

Partners Against Pain. Provides news
updates, pain control guides for patients,
support groups, and information, related
to pain management
www.partnersagainstpain.com

People Living With Cancer,
American Society of Clinical Oncology
www.plwc.org

Quackwatch. A nonprofit corporation
whose purpose is to combat health related
frauds, myths, fads, and fallacies
www.quackwatch.com

MEDICATION AND DIETARY SUPPLEMENT RECORD

Medications

Start Date	Brand Name	Generic Name	Dose/Amount	How Often	Stop Date

Dietary Supplements

Start Date	Supplement Name	Dose/Amount	How Often	Stop Date

Moderate and Simple Lifestyle Changes for Potential Prostate Cancer and Cardiovascular Risk Reduction

Lifestyle Change	Recommendation
Getting a cardiovascular disease risk assessment from your physician should be made a priority.	Know your lipid and blood pressure numbers as well as knowing your PSA values.
Maintain a healthy body weight.	A BMI or weight-to-height ratio should be part of your clinical record.
Choose from various weight-loss programs, if necessary. (Ask your physician first.)	Let the program fit your lifestyle and personality, but be sure to be monitored by your physician.
Replace saturated, trans-fatty acids and cholesterol with unsaturated fat.	Total fat intake may be less important than the *type* of fat you consume. Commercial plant sterols/stanols (in margarine and orange juice) may reduce your cholesterol.
Consume dietary fiber, especially soluble fiber.	You should aim for 10–25 grams/day of fiber each day. This comes from many products and can reduce your risk for several health problems.
Consume a variety of fruits and vegetables every day. (This doesn't limit you to tomato products.)	Eating lots of fruits and vegetables will expose you to numerous anti-cancer and anti-cardiovascular compounds.
Consume moderate amounts of traditional dietary soy and other "plant estrogen" products, such as ground flaxseed.	25 grams/day of soy protein and 1–2 tablespoons of ground flaxseed may improve lipid profiles and reduce your risk for numerous health conditions.
Consume moderate weekly intakes of canned (in water), broiled, baked, and raw—but not fried—fish, and other healthy sources of omega-3 fatty acids (example: nuts and cooking oils), dietary Vitamin D, Vitamin E, and selenium.	Several servings of fish weekly and a variety of nuts and cooking oils (example: soybean, canola, olive) provide various nutrients and reduce the risk of a cardiovascular event and other adverse health conditions.
Perform physical activity for at least 30 minutes every day, and lift weights or perform resistance exercises several times a week.	Aerobic and resistance exercise should be equally emphasized; both improve cardiovascular health, increase bone mineral density, reduce obesity, increase insulin sensitivity, and reduce the risk of cancer.
Don't smoke or drink alcohol in excess, and try to reduce the stress in your life.	Smoking, drinking, and stress are all risk factors for heart disease and certain cancers. These changes should be given as much attention as other lifestyle changes.

Questions to Ask Your Doctors

_____

_____

_____

_____

_____

_____

_____

_____

_____

_____

_____

_____

_____

_____

_____

_____

_____

_____

_____

_____

_____

_____

Questions to Ask Your Doctors

_____

_____

_____

_____

_____

_____

_____

_____

_____

_____

_____

_____

_____

_____

_____

_____

_____

_____

_____